MW01038266

DOCTORED DRAWINGS

ALSO BY MARK PODWAL

The Decline and Fall of the American Empire
Freud's da Vinci
A Book of Hebrew Letters
A Jewish Bestiary
The Book of Tens
Golem: A Giant Made of Mud
The Menorah Story
A Sweet Year
Jerusalem Sky: Stars, Crosses and Crescents

ILLUSTRATED BY MARK PODWAL

The Golem (by Elie Wiesel)
Six Days of Destruction (by Elie Wiesel)
A Passover Haggadah (by Elie Wiesel)
Dybbuk: A Story Made in Heaven (by Francine Prose)
Jewish Days (by Francine Klagsbrun)
The Angel's Mistake: Stories of Chelm (by Francine Prose)
You Never Know: A Legend of the Lamed-vavniks (by Francine Prose)
Moses and the Angels (by Ileene Smith Sobel)
King Solomon and His Magic Ring (by Elie Wiesel)
The Demons' Mistake: A Story from Chelm (by Francine Prose)
Fallen Angels (by Harold Bloom)

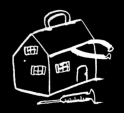

DOCTORED
DRAWINGS

MARK PODWAL

BELLEVUE LITERARY PRESS

New York

First published in the United States in 2007 by
Bellevue Literary Press
New York

FOR INFORMATION ADDRESS:
Bellevue Literary Press
NYU School of Medicine
550 First Avenue
OBV 640
New York, NY 10016

PICTURE CREDITS

*Many of these drawings first appeared on the OP-ED page of The New York Times. Drawings on p. 32 New York
University Medical Quarterly; pp. 34, 35 Dermatopathology: Practical and Conceptual; pp. 42, 43, 44
Journal of Dermatological Surgery; pp. 56, 57, 58, 59, 60, 61, 62, 63 first published in Freud's da Vinci,
Images Graphique, 1977; p. 71 The Wall Street Journal; p. 82 Hadassah Magazine.*

This book was published with the generous support of
Bellevue Literary Press's founding donor the Arnold Simon Family Trust
and the Bernard & Irene Schwartz Foundation.

Cataloging-in-Publication Data is available from the Library of Congress.

Book design and type formatting by Bernard Schleifer
Manufactured in the United States of America
ISBN-13 978-1-934137-02-4 / ISBN-10 1-934137-02-4
FIRST EDITION
1 3 5 7 9 8 6 4 2

In memory of
Saul Farber, M.D.

INTRODUCTION

It takes a doctor who's partly somewhere else to be able to look at his own profession from the outside.

When I first met Mark Podwal, when we were in the same class at the New York University School of Medicine in the late 1960s, he was already partly somewhere else. Even as he studied medicine he was an artist. Even as he learned to treat patients he grew in his mastery of drawing and illustration. He had a great talent in the first field, and no less a talent in the second.

And, since then, he has lived in both worlds. He has continued to practice dermatology as well as develop his gifts as an artist. For three decades, readers of the *New York Times* and other publications, as well as those who have seen his art in numerous books and exhibitions, have been illuminated by his interpretation of messages—political, historical, mythical, religious.

Of the many realms he has touched with his artistic work, two stand out as drawing him back to them time and again.

One is the realm of Jewish tradition, which infused him with its images and which he has infused in turn with his.

The other is the realm of medicine, which also infused him with its images, and which has also been infused with his.

By chance, Podwal's work in art, and mine in writing, intersected twice in the *New York Times.* In 1994 I discovered that an essay of mine on the dangers of physician-assisted suicide, titled "First Do No Harm," was illustrated by a stark drawing of a skeletal hand whose fingers had been transformed into surgical instruments: the hand that could heal but also harm. It conveyed my argument better than my words did. And in 2002 an essay of mine in the *Times,* titled "Appropriating the Holocaust," was illustrated by a striking Podwal image of multiple train tracks, in the shape of a swastika, leading to the *anus mundi* that was Auschwitz.

But most of Podwal's work hasn't focused on death and destruction. In the realm of medical themes, in fact, it has been, in the main, very different—imaginative, clarifying, iconoclastic, incisive, whimsical, absurd, funny. It took a doctor to be able to turn doctors, including himself, into caricatured specialists, each identified by an instrument— surgical, say, or dermatological, or gynecological—typically used by that specialty. It took a doctor to be able to summarize cancer as a cell that had turned into a crab— the astrological cancer. It took a doctor to be able to understand the complexity of an intensive care unit, but also to understand its inescapably embedded costs.

For Podwal, growths, with which he deals every day as a physician, could also be seen as blooming flowers. For him, the idea of radical surgery could be, whimsically, applied to hair transplants, which are, in the version radicalized by his imagination, inserted not into the scalp but into the brain below. A second opinion in the age of rationed care is not a second stethoscope listening to the patient but a second stethoscope listening to the first. The complexity and specificity of medical treatments are captured in a drawing purporting to teach which pills or injections treat which ills at which site in the body. The consequences of war are evoked by a bone dangling from a military ribbon. The projection of government, through Medicare, into the lives of all Americans is shown by a Capitol dome sprouting tentacles that hold medical instruments. Medical conditions, seen under a microscope, reify their metaphorical medical names: ichthyosis (fish skin), drawn at high power resolution, reveals—little fish! And dermatophytosis (a fungal infection), as seen through

Podwal's microscope, reveals—what else?—mushrooms. Only a doctor—and a dermatologist at that—would have the authority needed to achieve such concretized whimsy.

Only a doctor, moreover, living in the age of managed care, which in some ways has ensnared not only patients but also physicians, could have the insight, provoked by bureaucratically-induced pain, to draw an image of a "provider"—as insurance companies and Medicare have come to call doctors—as a voodoo doll: white-coated, impaled by syringes, in managed-care agony. In fact, the idea of managed care as a medical process that doesn't work—because it maims the doctor, the patient or medical care itself—is evoked more than once, as in the drawing of a Rube Goldberg-like medical system that managed care has managed to bury in the morass of its own complexity.

Mark Podwal has a lot to say about medicine. And he says it with authority, sincerity, gravity and humor—and from the outside no less than from the inside.

—WALTER REICH, M.D.

Yitzhak Rabin Memorial Professor of International Affairs, Ethics and Human Behavior, and Professor of Psychiatry and Behavioral Science, George Washington University; Senior Scholar, Woodrow Wilson Center; and former director, United States Holocaust Memorial Museum.

DOCTORED DRAWINGS

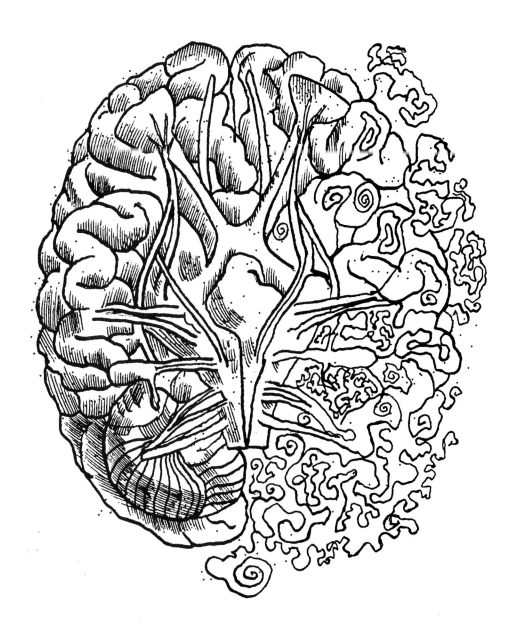

ALZHEIMER'S

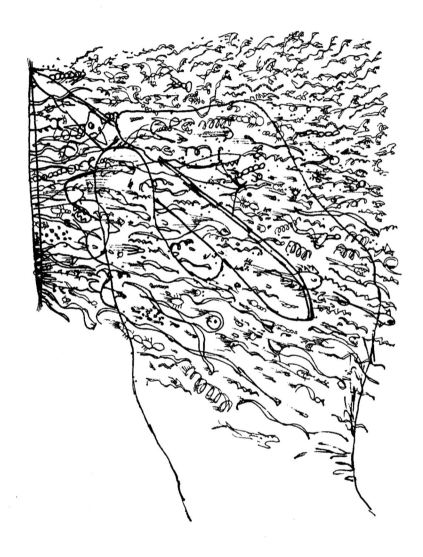

DISEASE

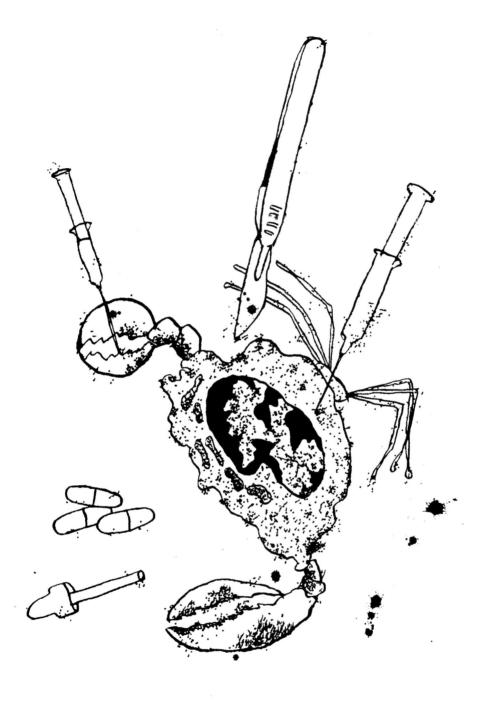

THE WAR AGAINST CANCER

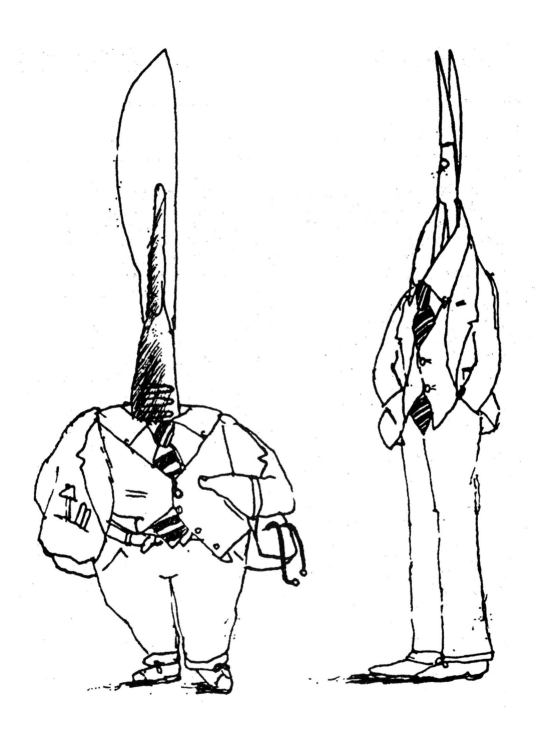

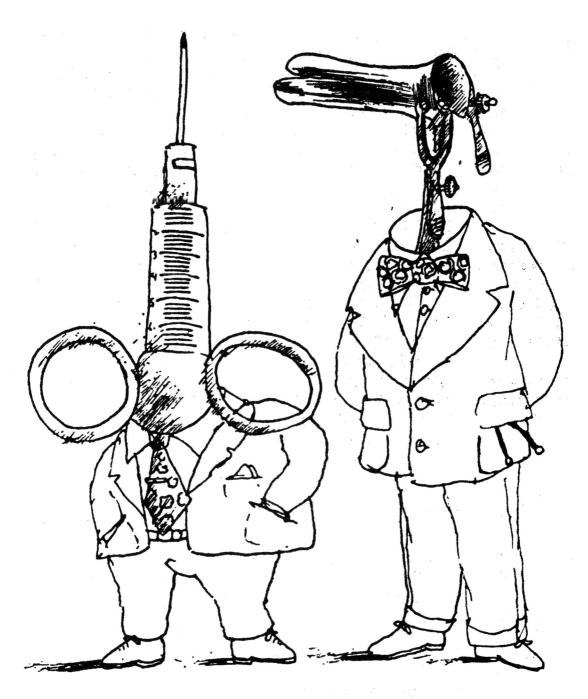

THE SPECIALISTS

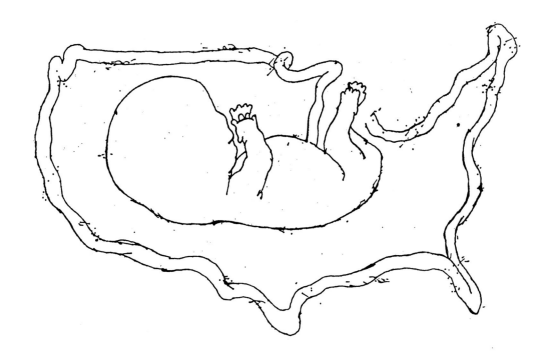

AN ABORTION

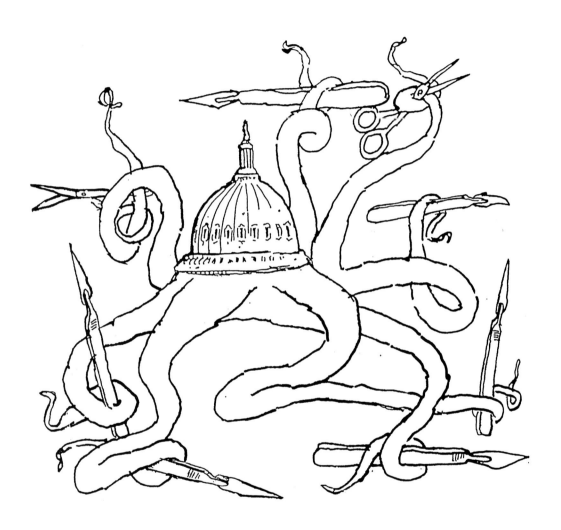

MEDISCARE

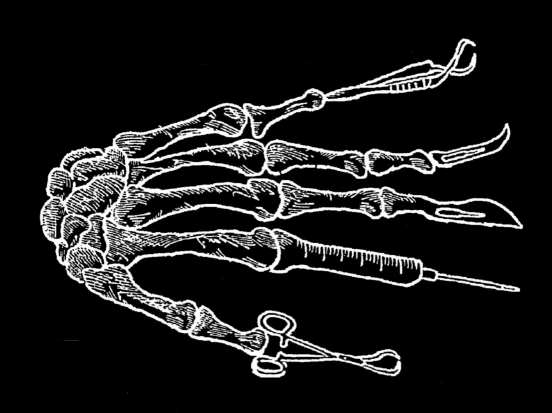

FIRST DO NO HARM

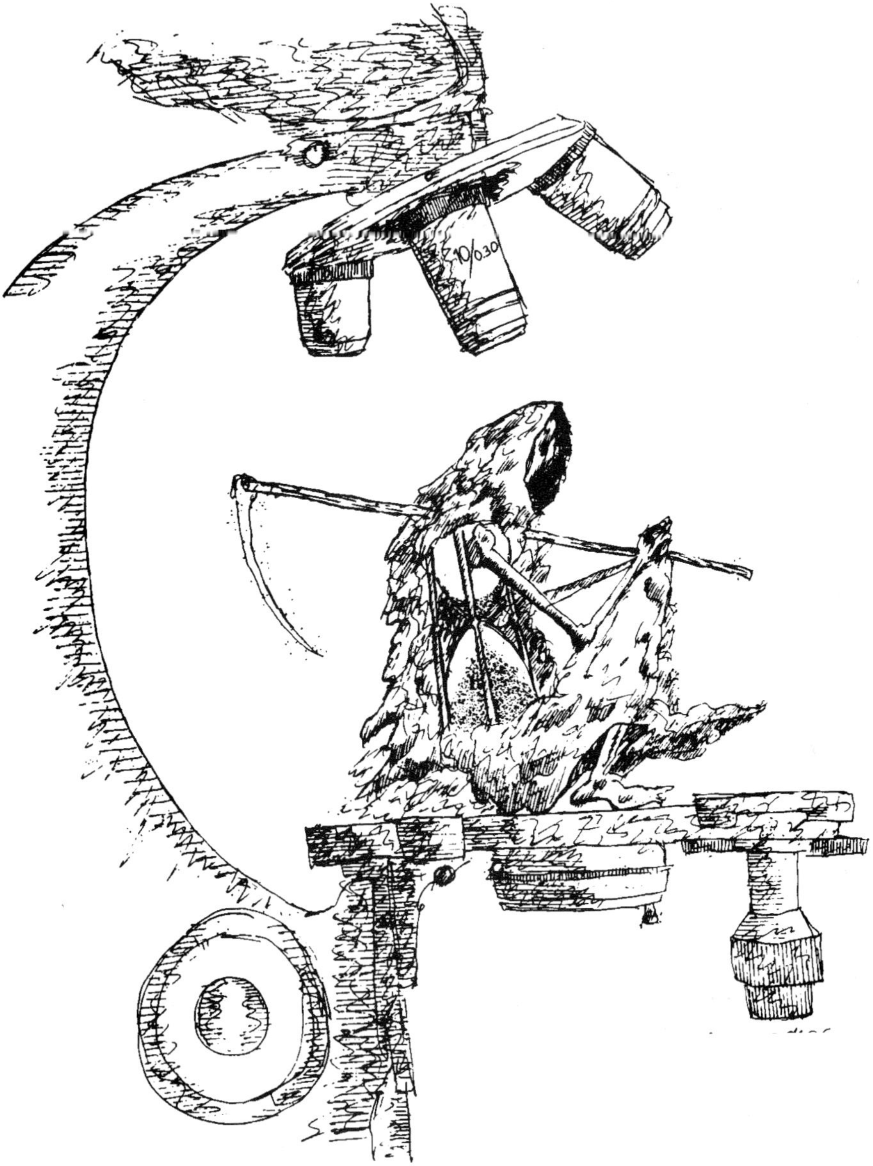
10/0.30

AIDS Research

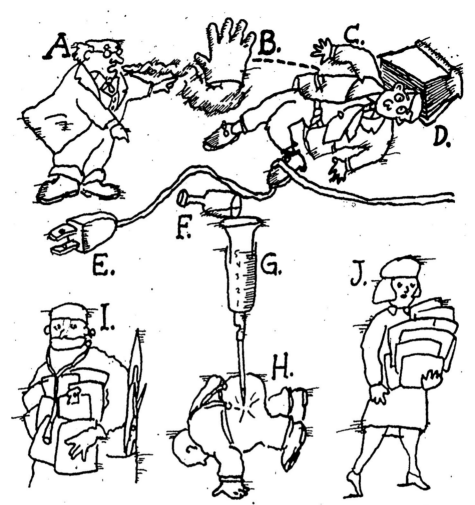

HOT AIR FROM SENATOR (A) FILLS LATEX EXAMINING GLOVE (B)
WHICH REACHES INTO POCKET OF SMALL BUSINESSMAN (C) STUNNED
WHEN 1300 PAGE HEALTHCARE PROPOSAL (D) HITS HIM AS HE TRIPS,
PULLING PLUG (E) FROM MAGNETIC RESONANCE IMAGING SCANNER
AND SPILLING TINY BOTTLE OF MALPRACTICE LAWYER'S SWEAT (F) WHICH
FALLS ON SYRINGE (G) THAT INJECTS PATIENT (H) WHILE
DOCTOR (I) AND NURSE (J) ARE BUSY WITH GOVERNMENT
GUIDELINES.   (APOLOGIES TO RUBE GOLDBERG)

CLINTON'S HEALTH PLAN

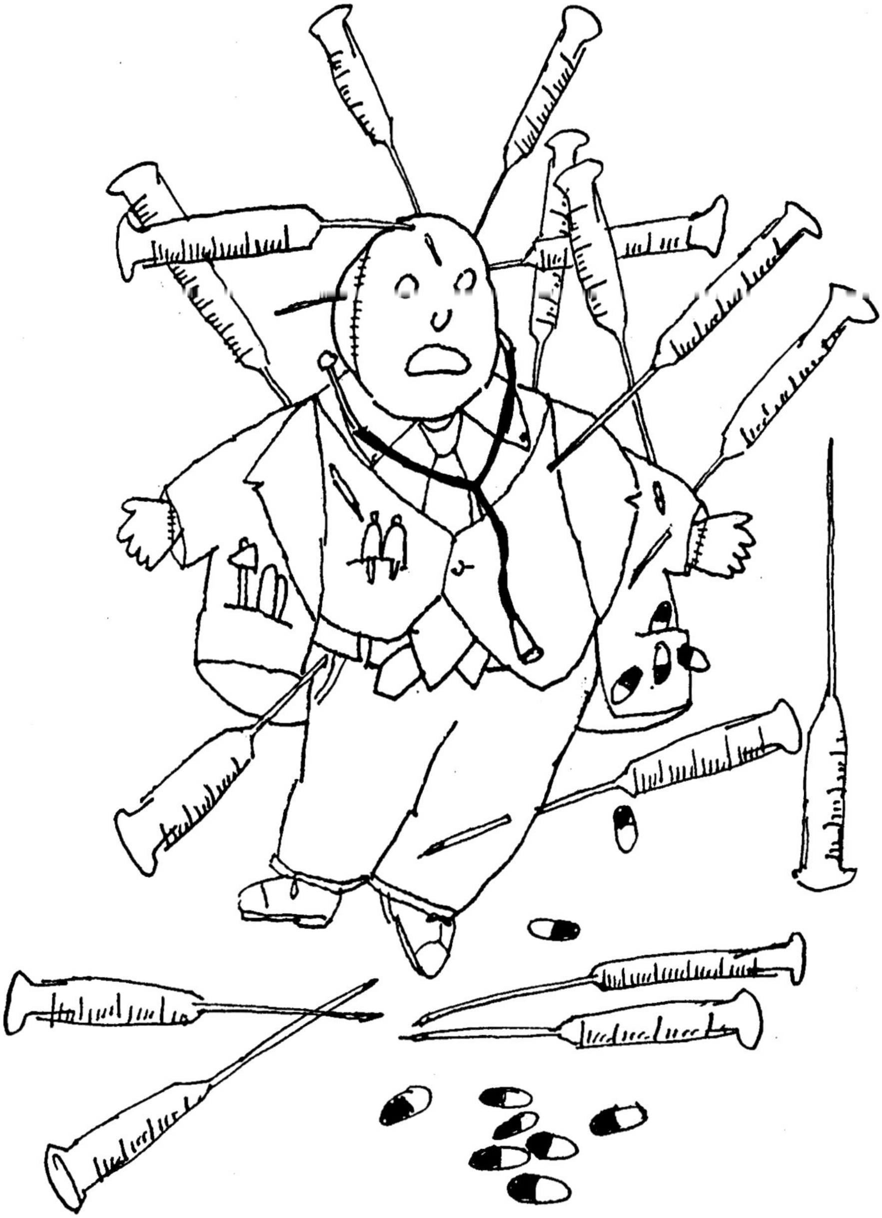

HMO Provider

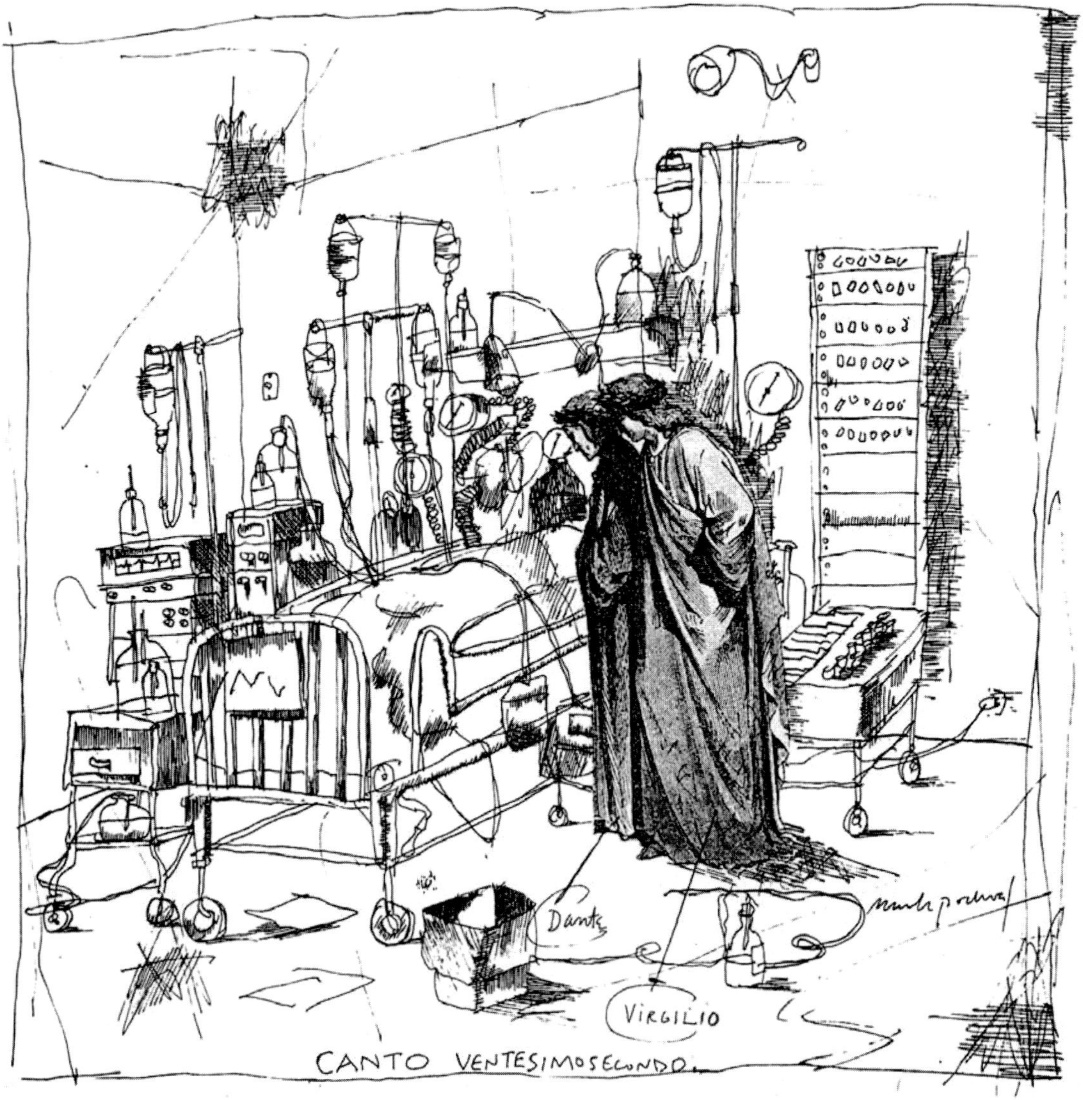
Dante
VIRGILIO
CANTO VENTESIMOSECONDO.

DANTE AND VIRGIL

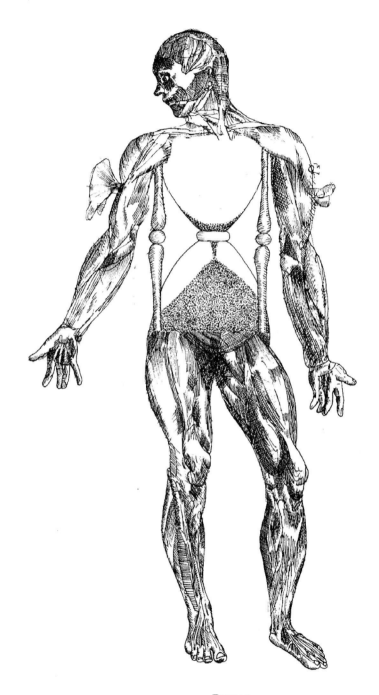

DYING

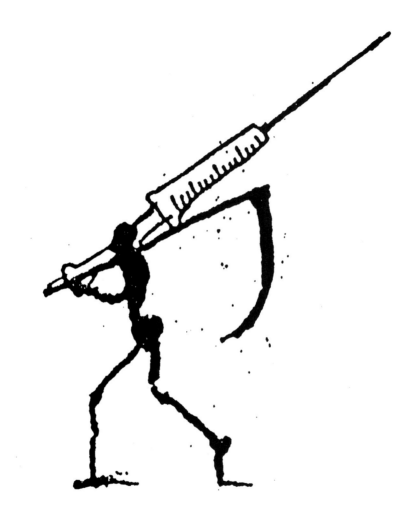

ANGEL OF DEATH

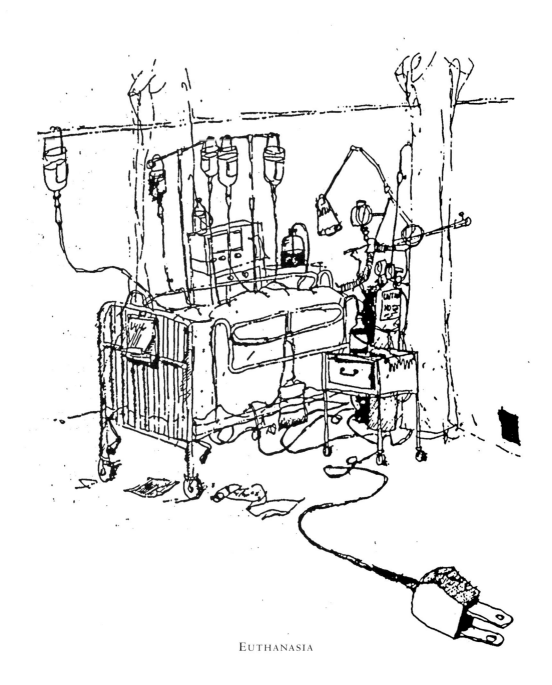

EUTHANASIA

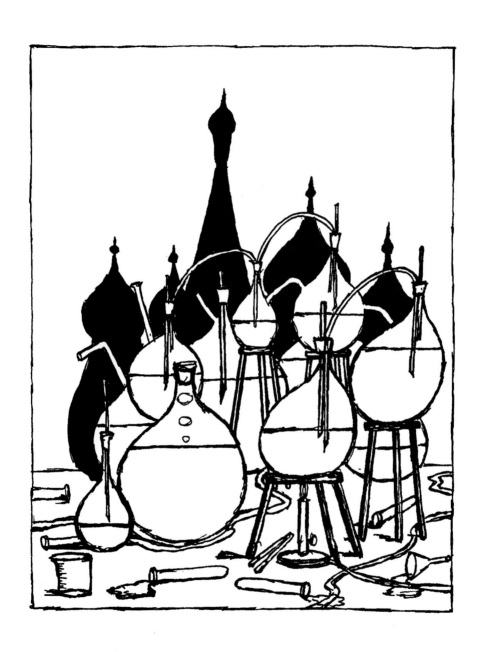

SOVIET ARSENAL

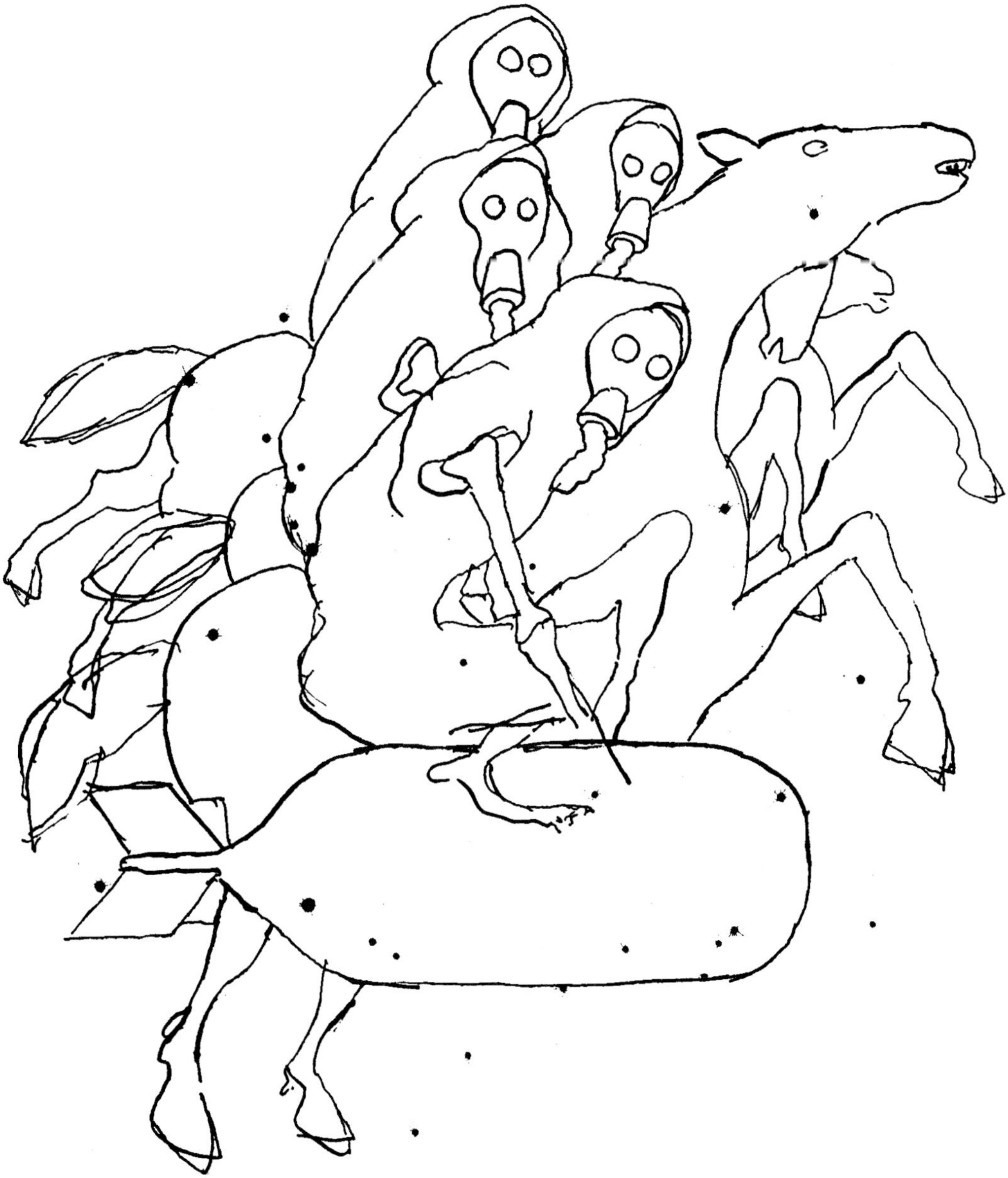

Nerve Gas

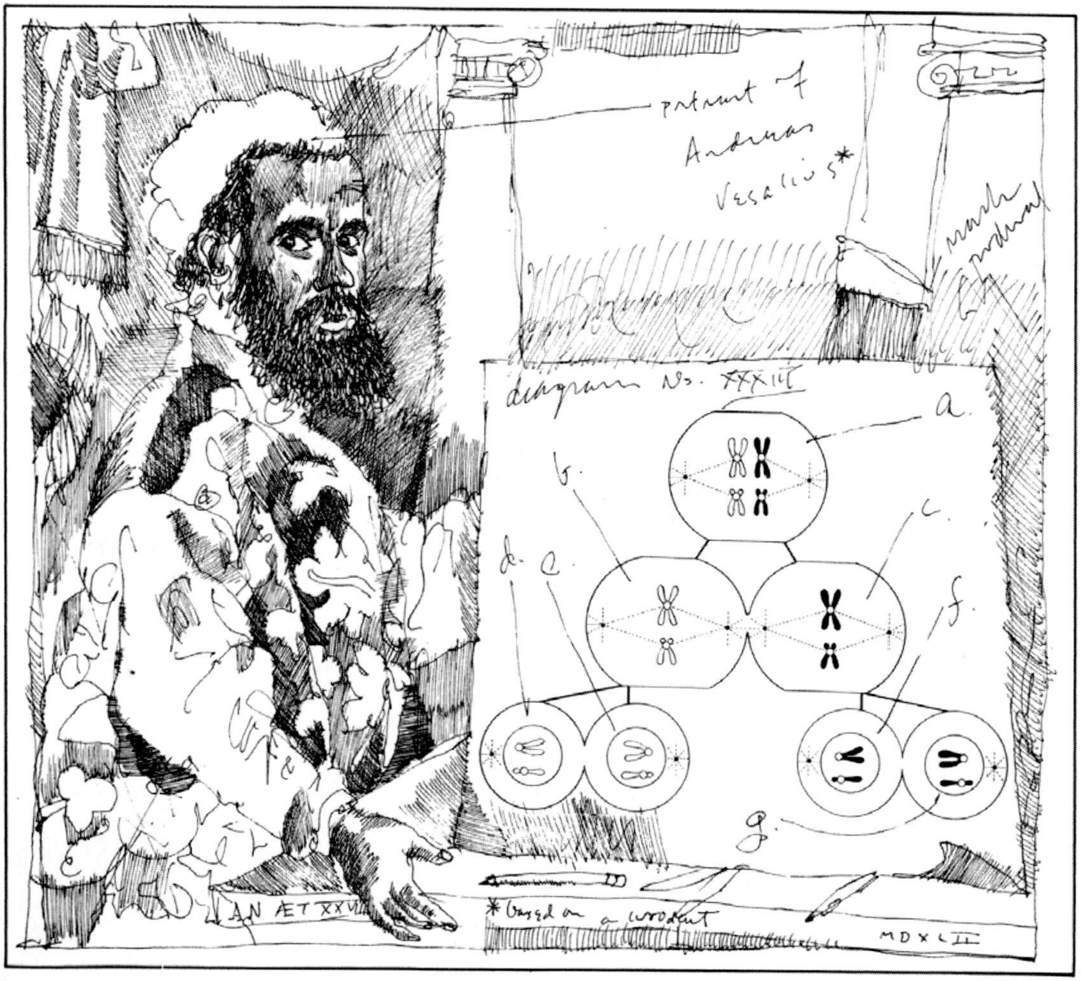
portrait of Andreas Vesalius*
diagram No. XXXIII
a.
b.
c.
d.
e.
f.
g.
*based on a woodcut
MDXLII

GENETICS

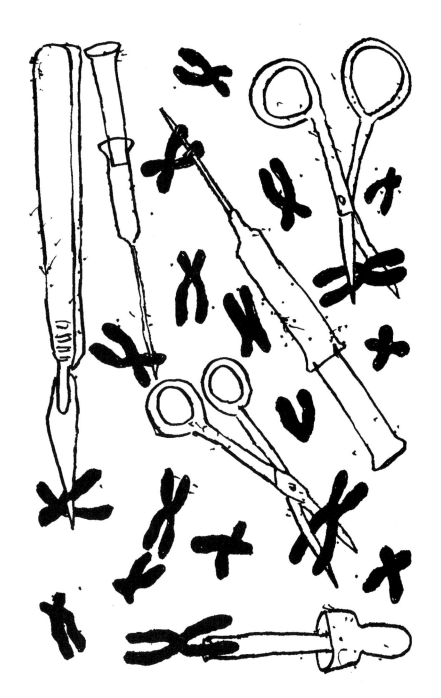

GENETIC ENGINEERING

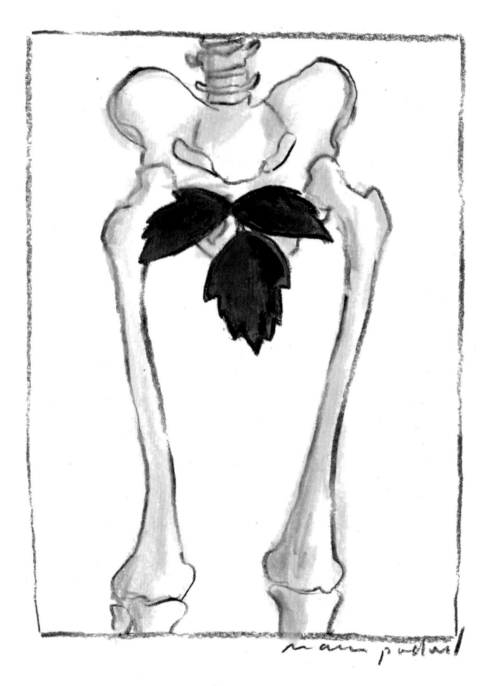

POISON IVY

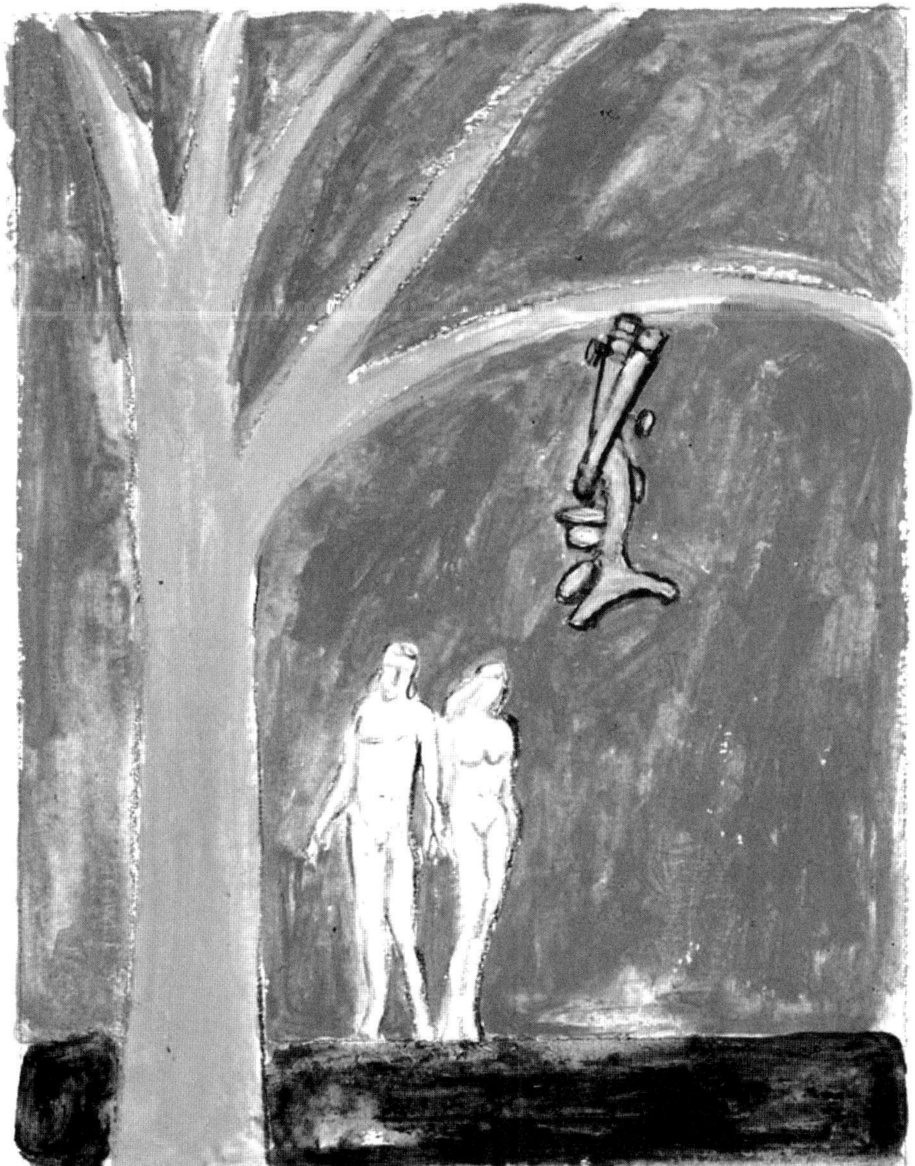

KNOWLEDGE

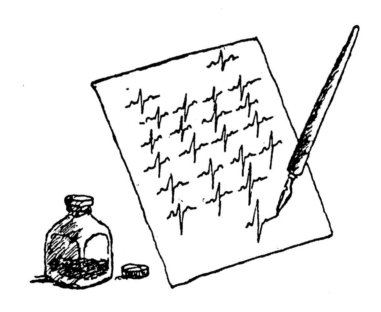

DOCTOR'S HANDWRITING

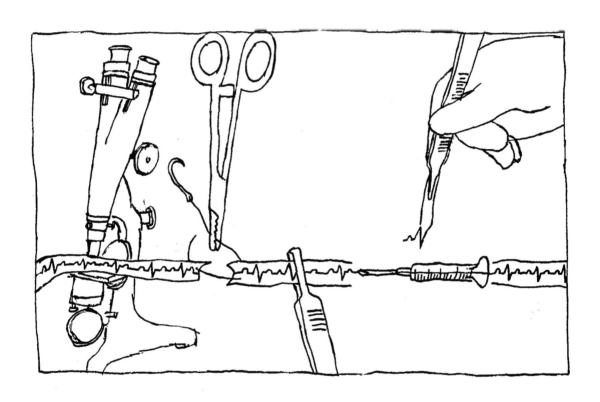

LIFELINE

A

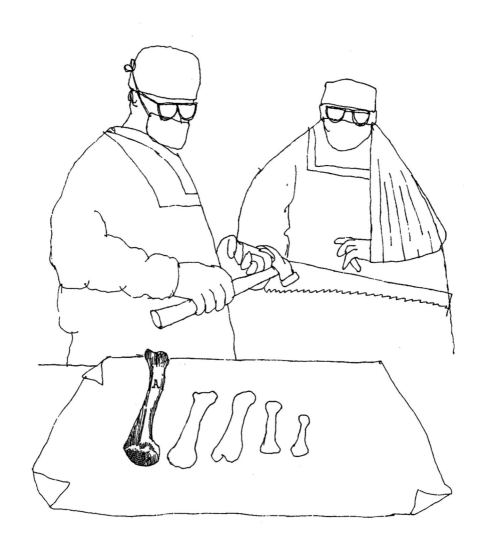

Orthopedists

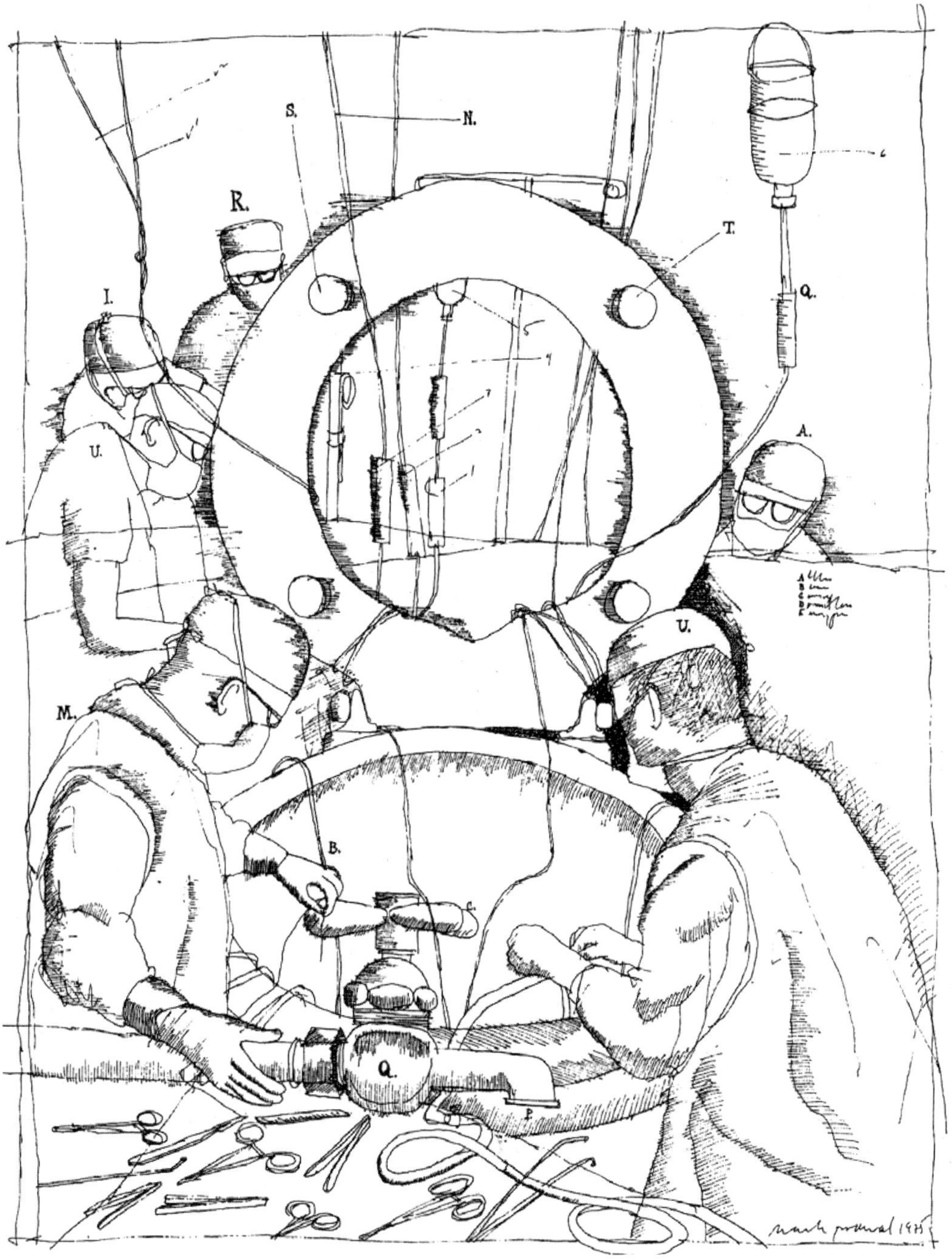
S.
N.
R.
T.
I.
Q.
U.
A.
U.
M.
B.
C.
Q.
P.

Urologists Operating in Their Field

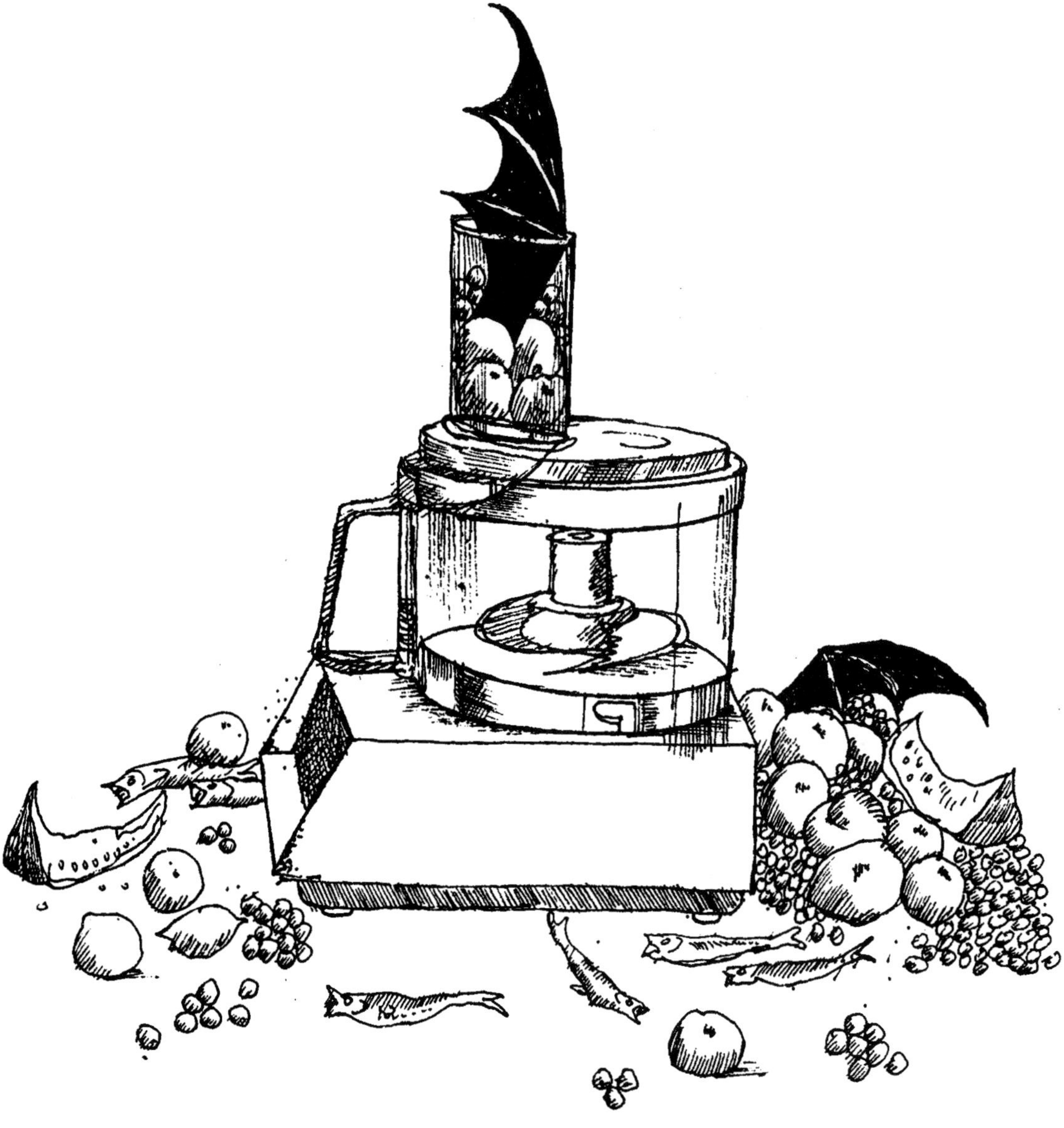

ALTERNATIVE MEDICINE

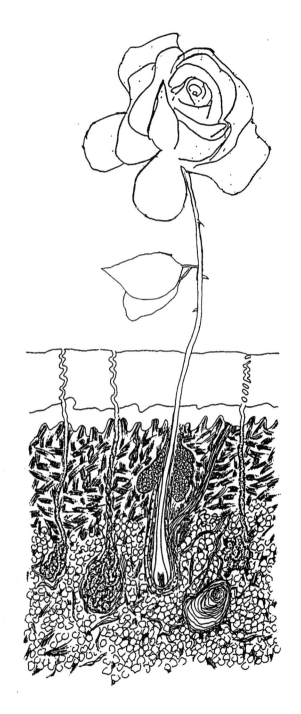

FLOWERING FOLLICLE

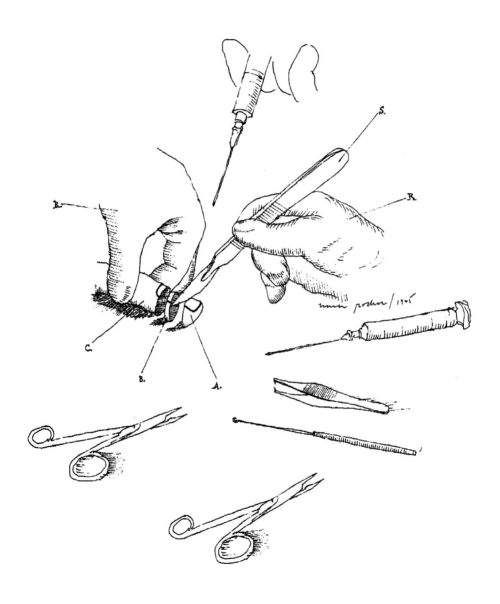

FINGERNAIL BIOPSY (POOR TECHNIQUE)

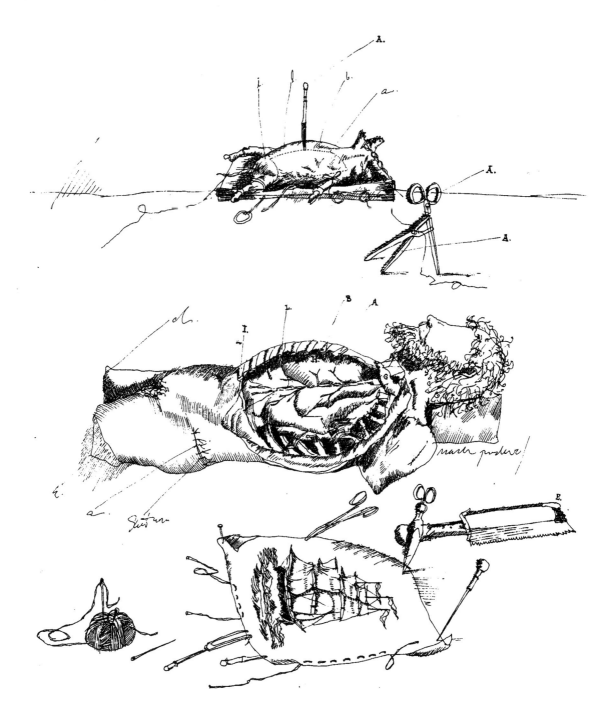

WIDE EXCISION AND GRAFT TECHNIQUE
FOR REMOVAL OF TATTOO

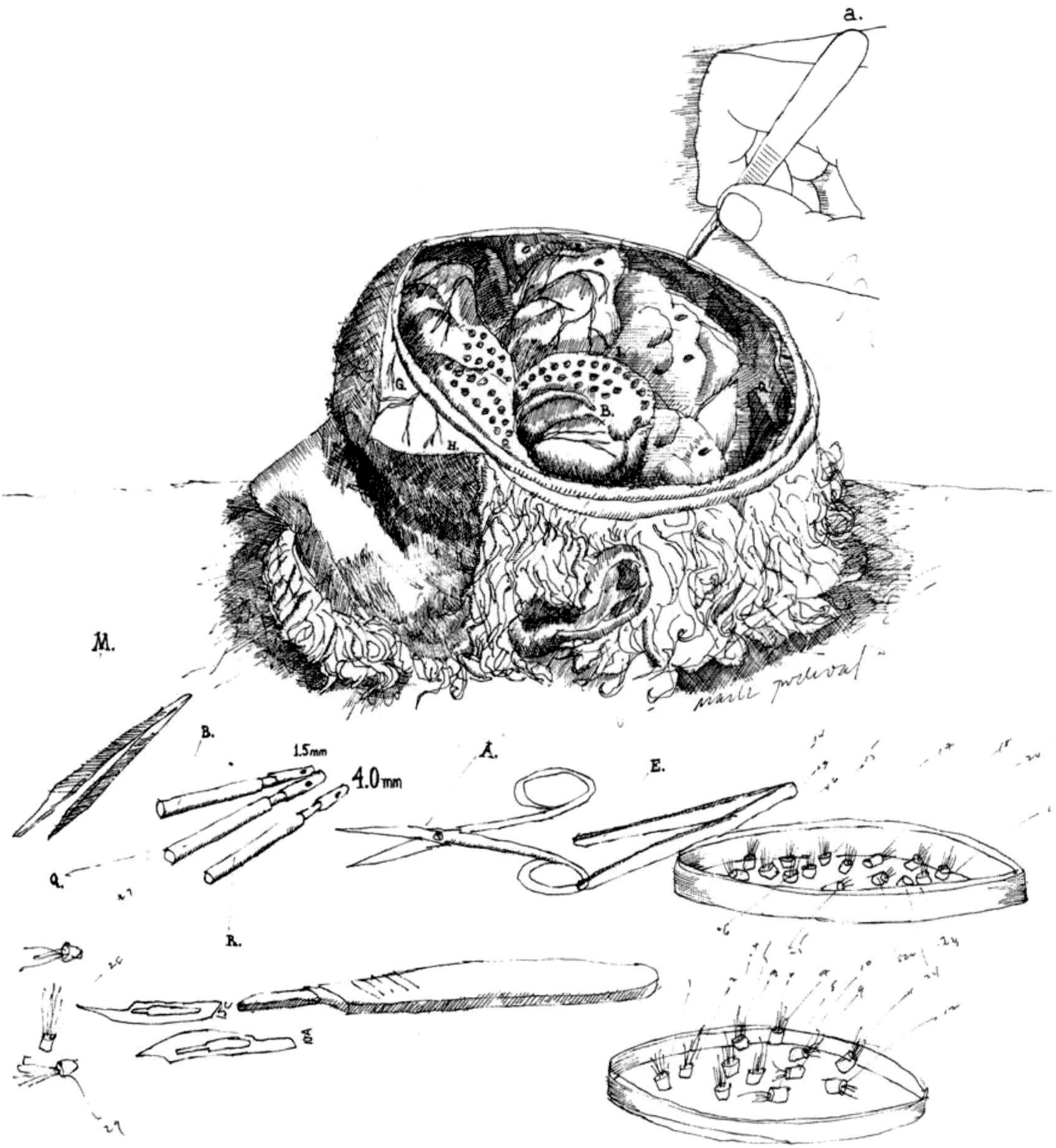
a.
B.
G.
H.
M.
B.
1.5mm
4.0mm
A.
E.
Q.
R.

Incorrect Hair Transplant Technique

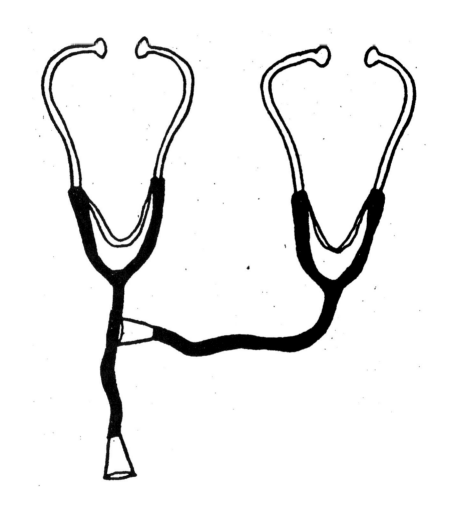

SECOND OPINION

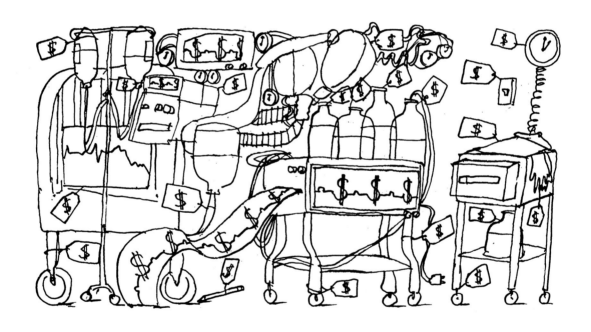

EXPENSIVE CARE UNIT

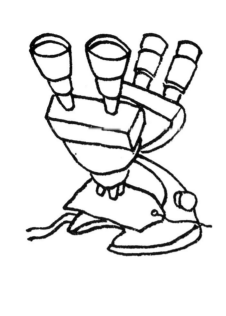

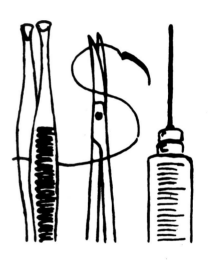

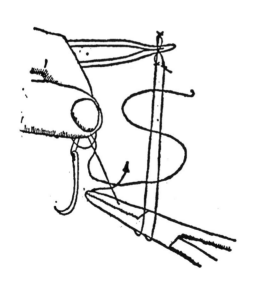

HEALTH COSTS

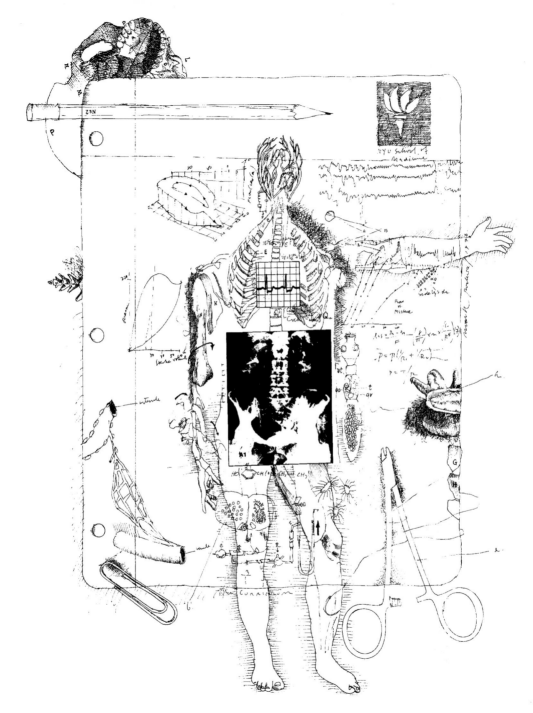

MEDICAL SCHOOL

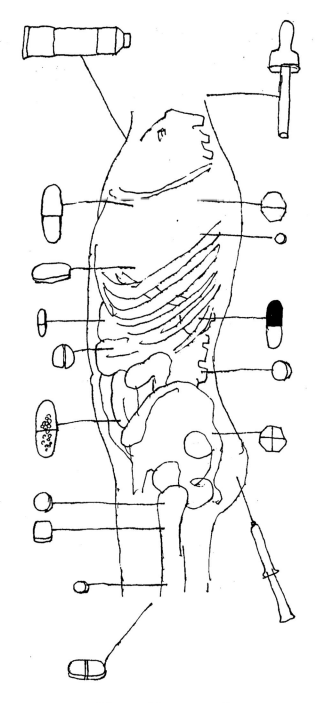

WHERE MEDICINES GO

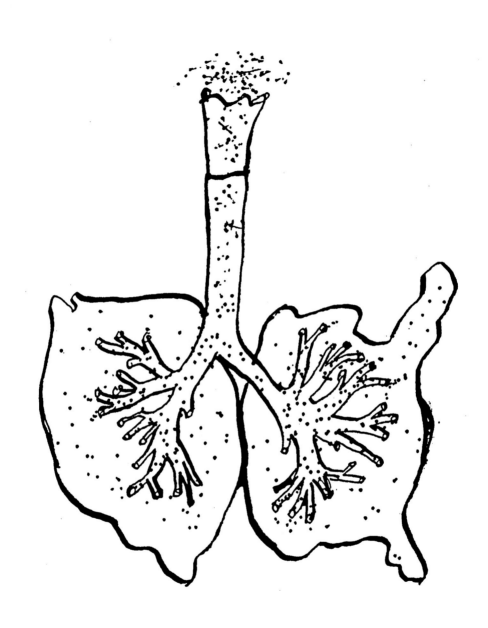

EPIDEMIC U.S.A.

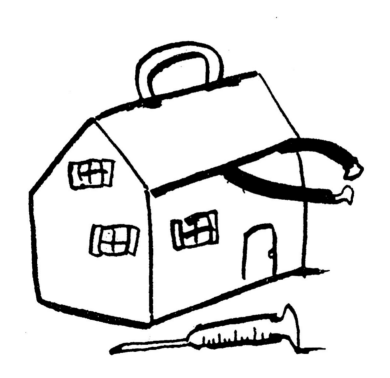

HOUSE CALL

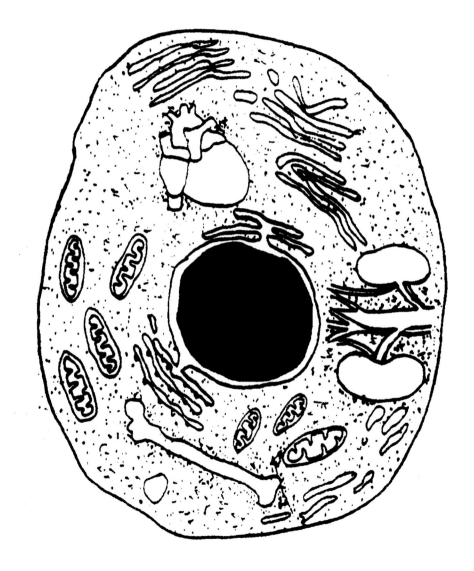

STEM CELL

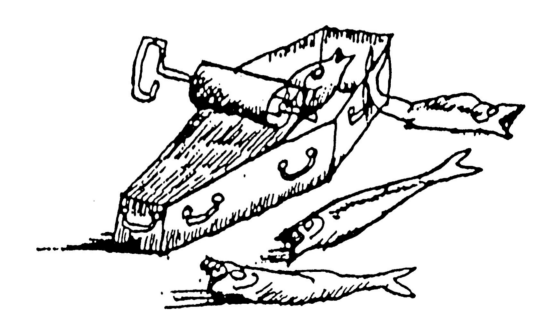

Omega-3

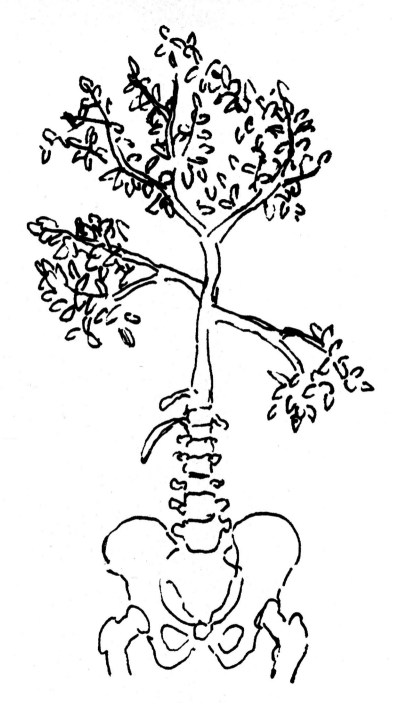

HUMAN NATURE

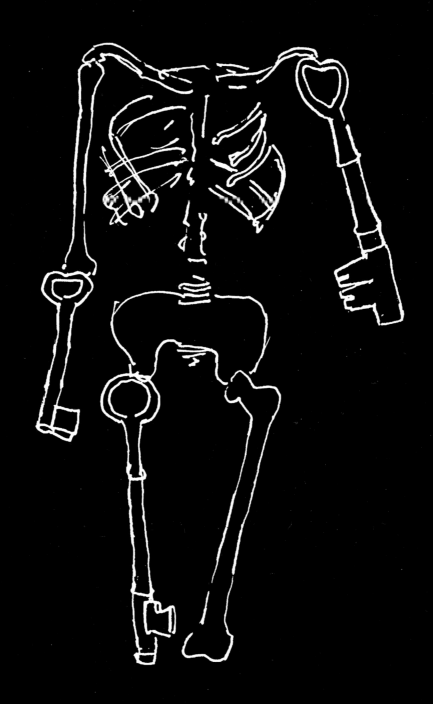

SKELETON KEYS

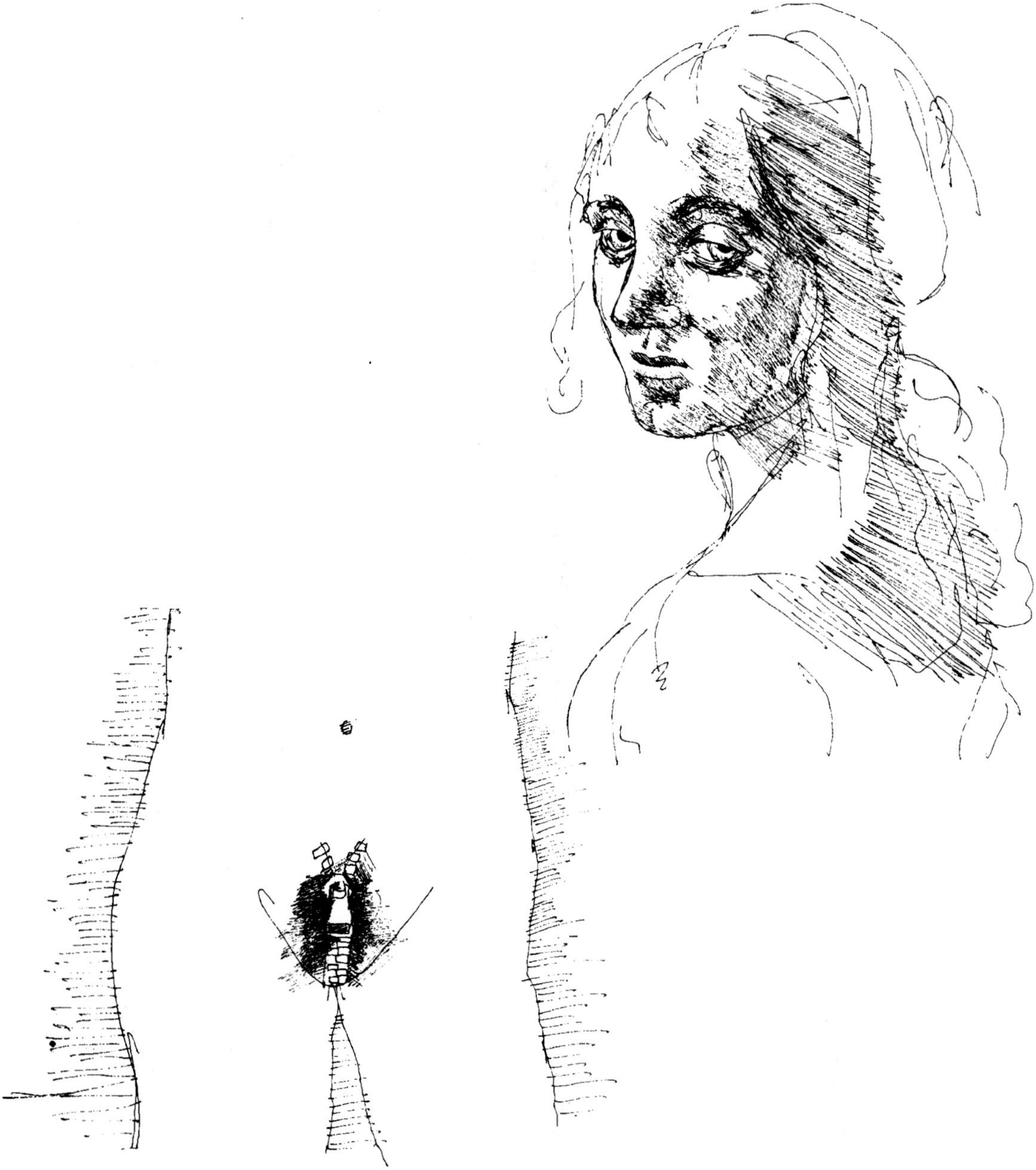

Study for *The Virgin of the Rocks*

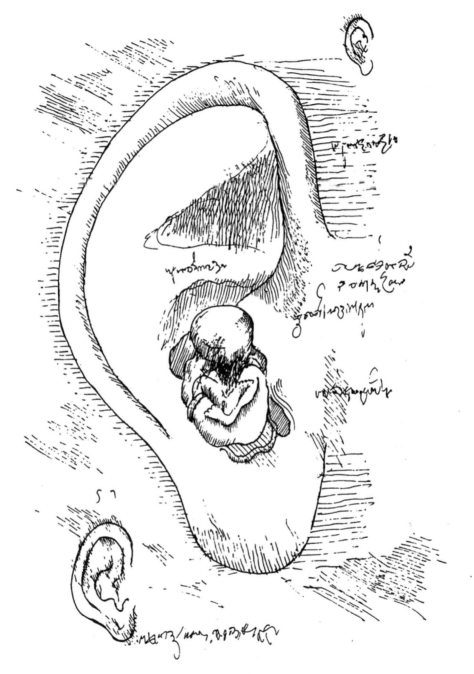

An Aural Fixation

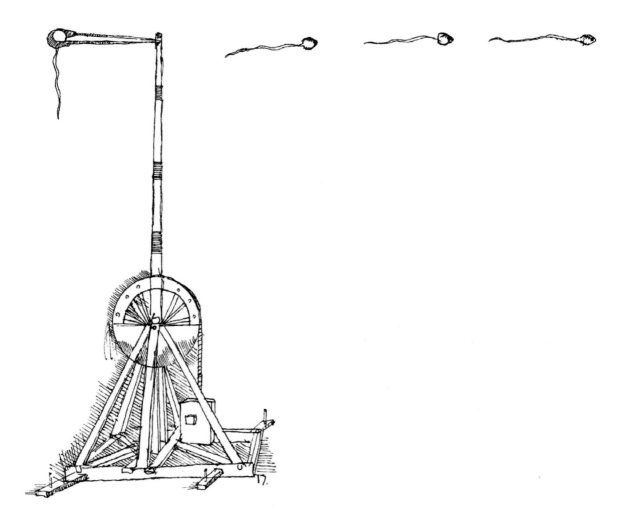

ARTIFICIAL INSEMINATION DEVICE

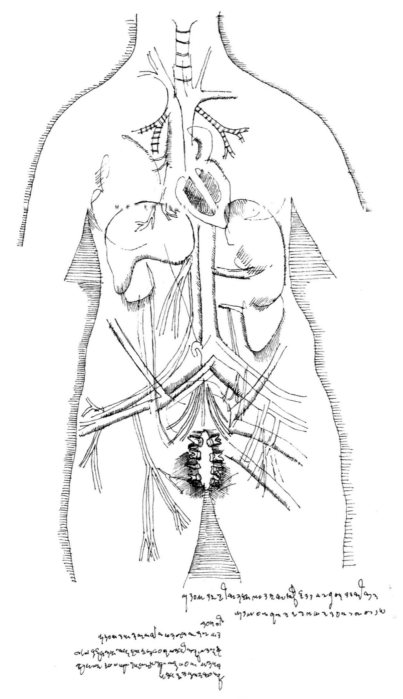

VAGINA WITH TEETH

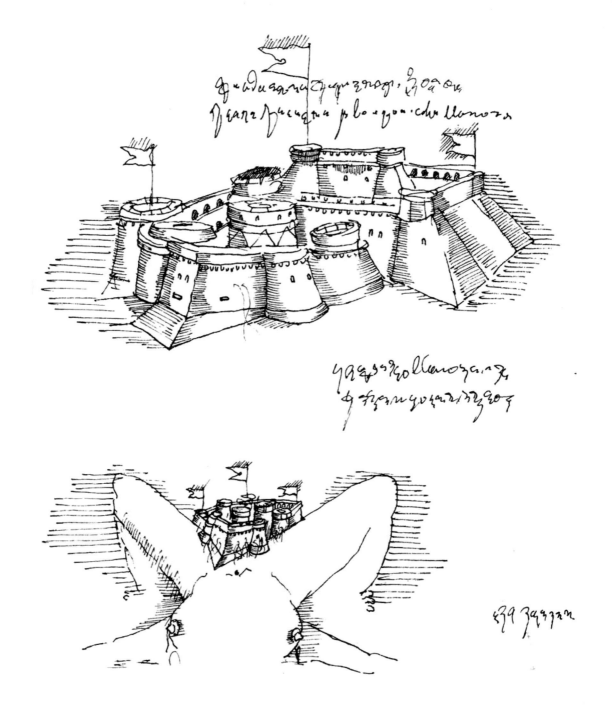

FORTIFICATION TO PREVENT THE SPREAD OF
VENEREAL DISEASE

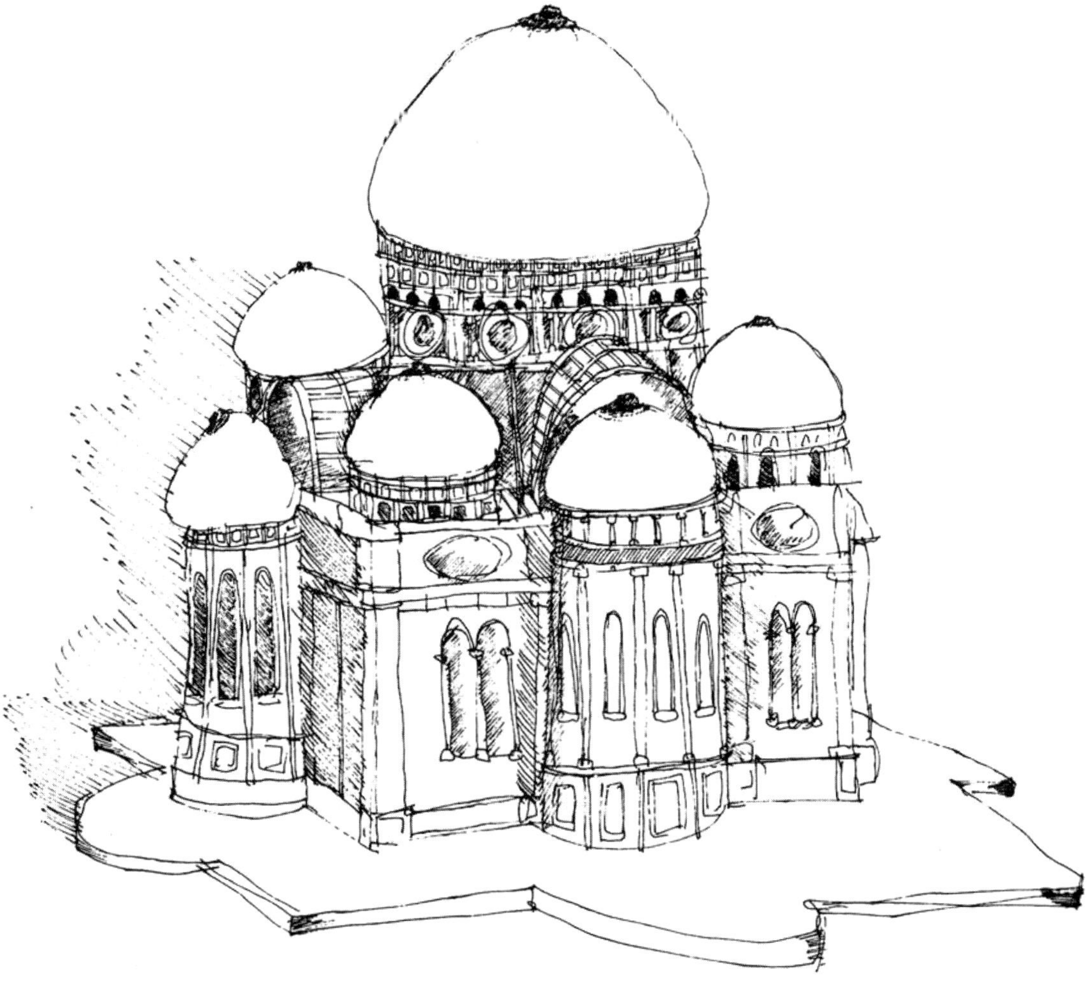

Church of Our Holy Mother

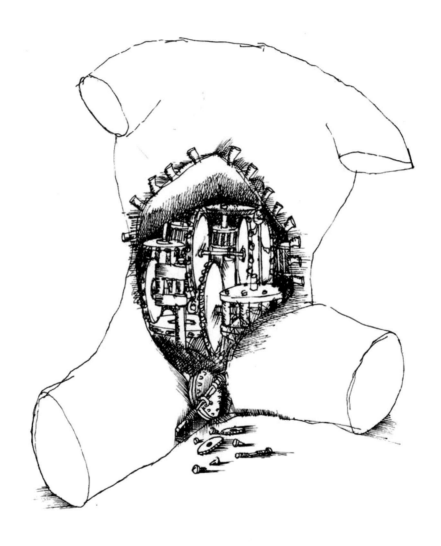

AUTOPSY STUDY

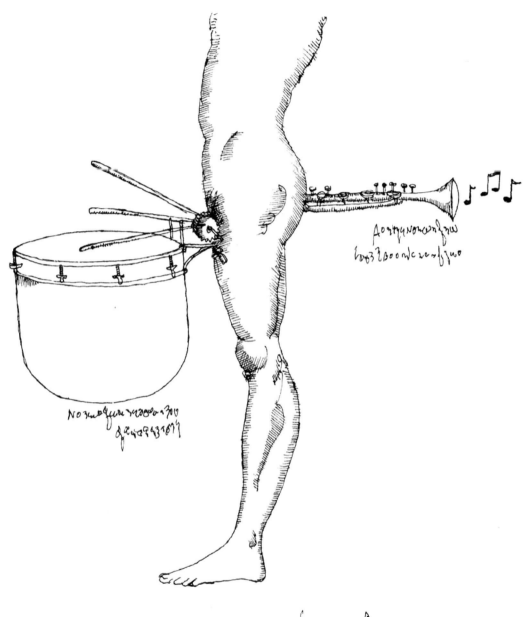

ONE MAN BAND

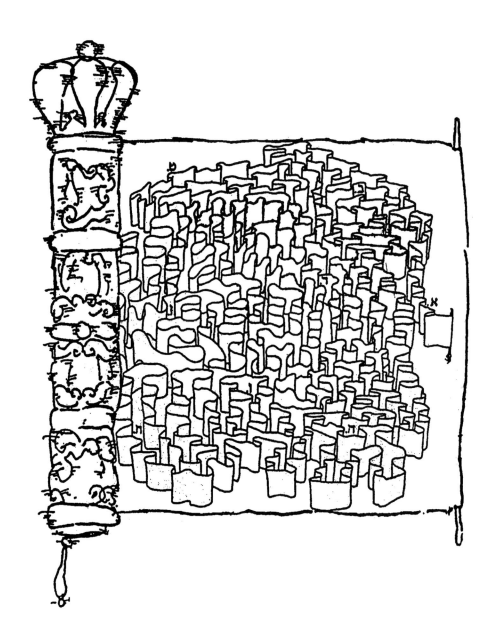

A MEGILLAH

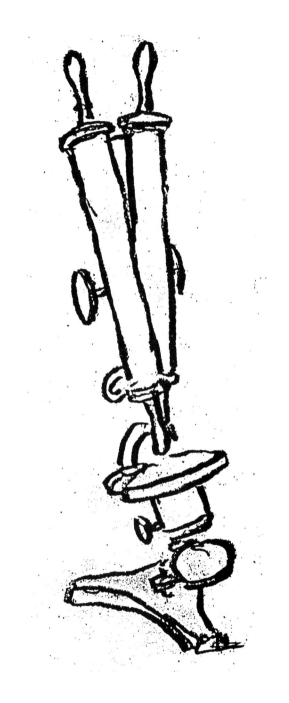

ON JEWISH MEDICAL ETHICS

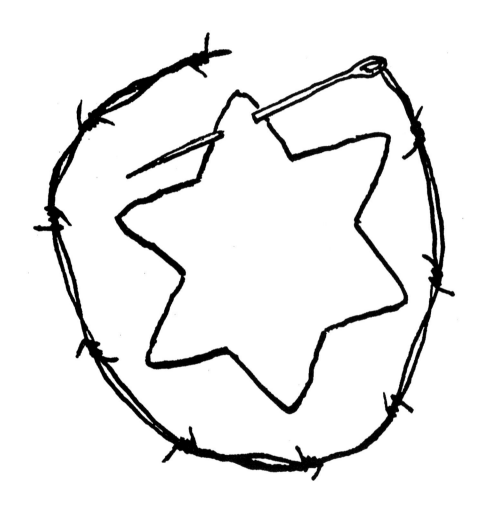

AUSCHWITZ

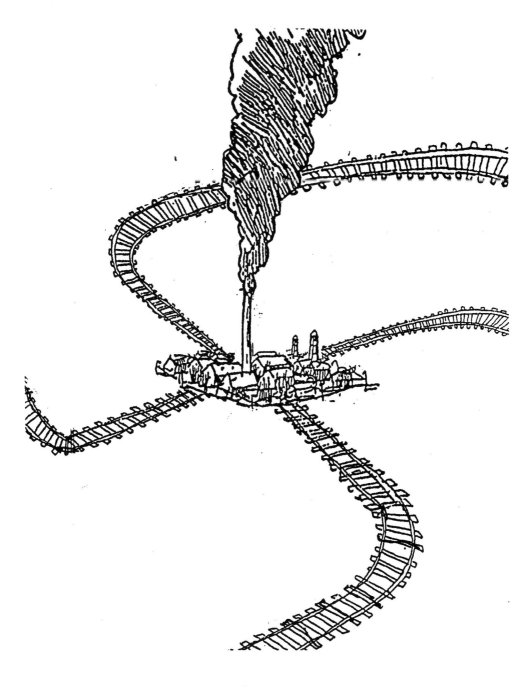

GENOCIDE

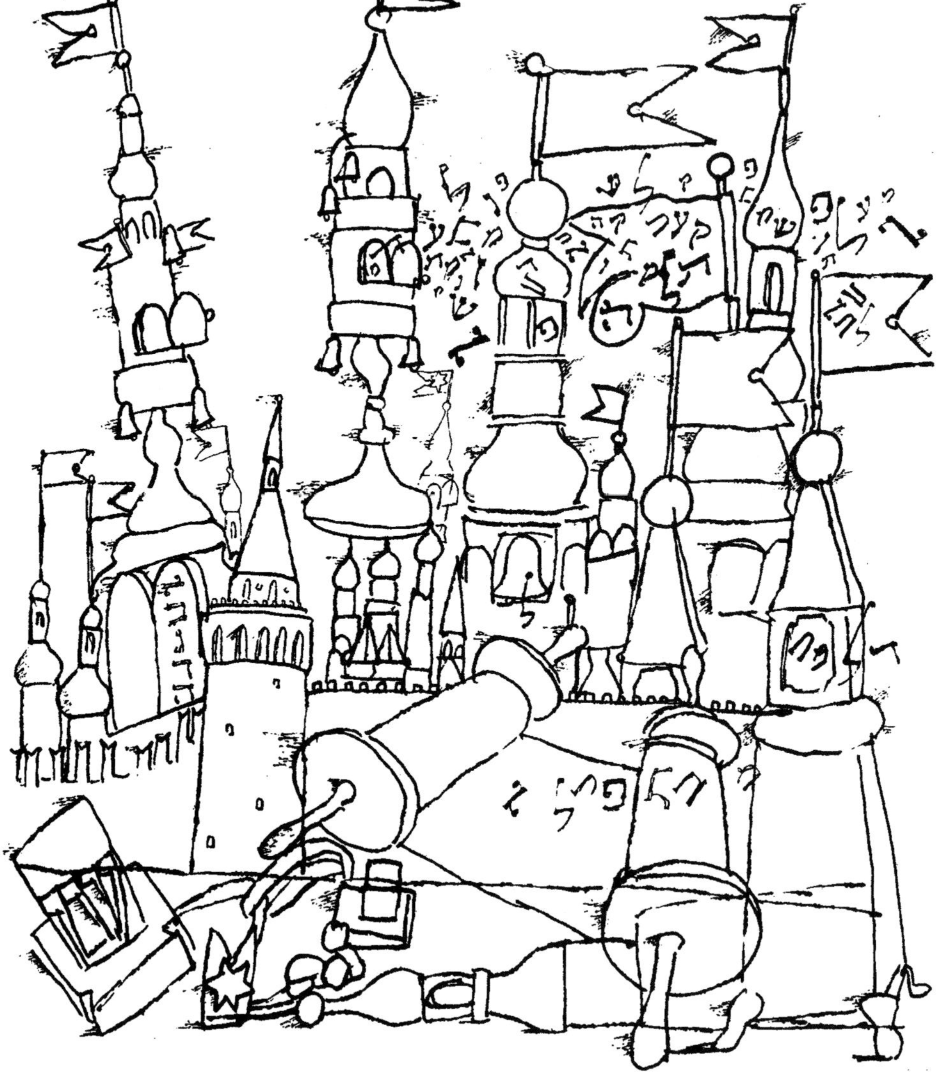

On Soviet Jewry

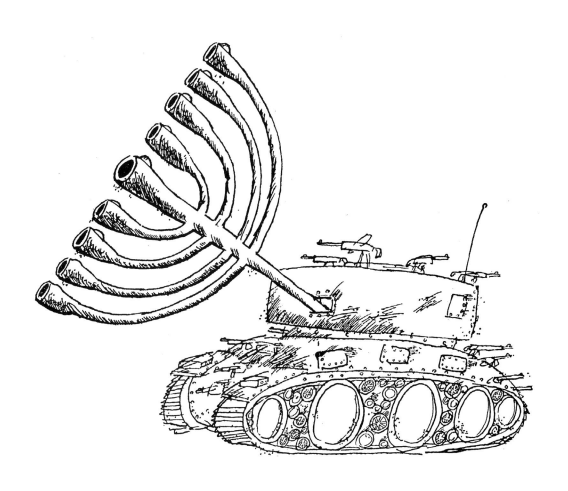

ISRAELI TANK

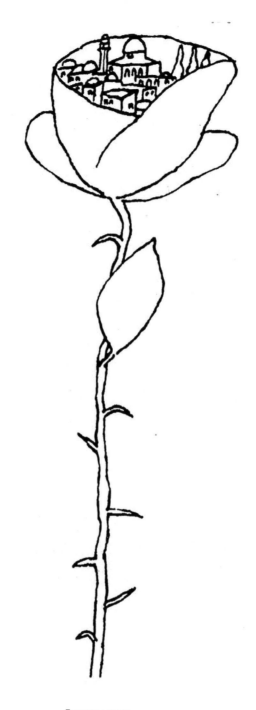

JERUSALEM

15
PALESTINE
15
ISRAEL
ישראל

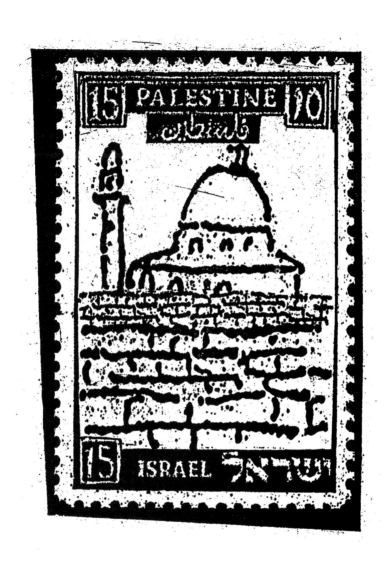

Jerusalem the Impossible Partition

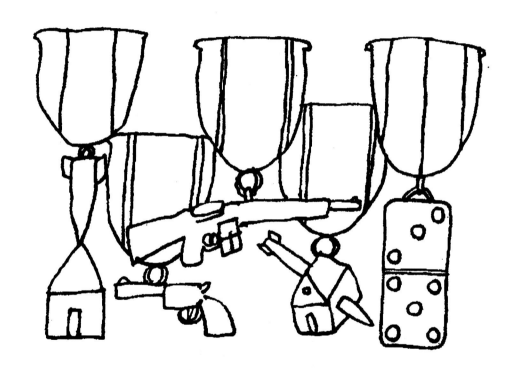

VIETNAM

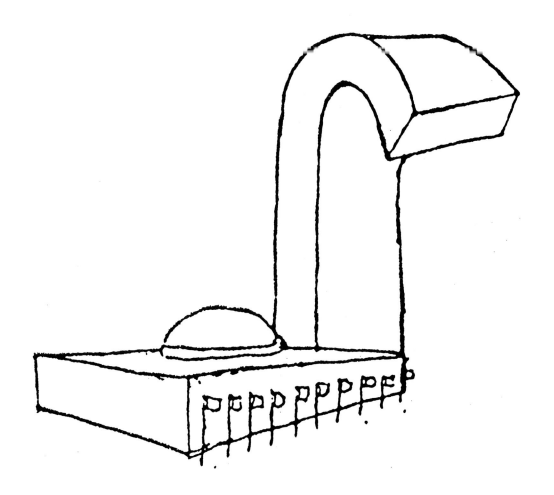

IMPOTENT

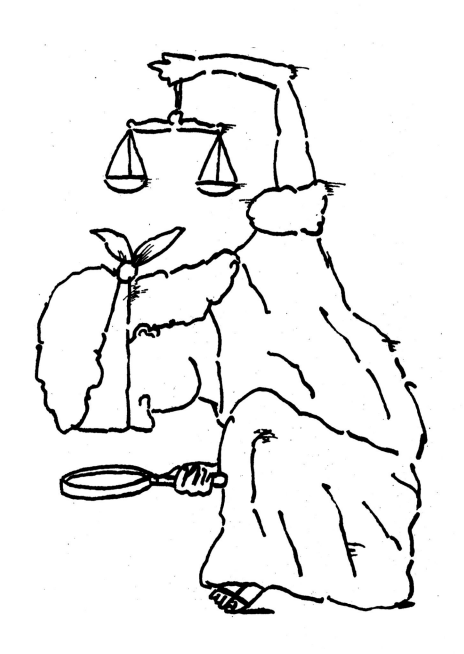

BLIND JUSTICE

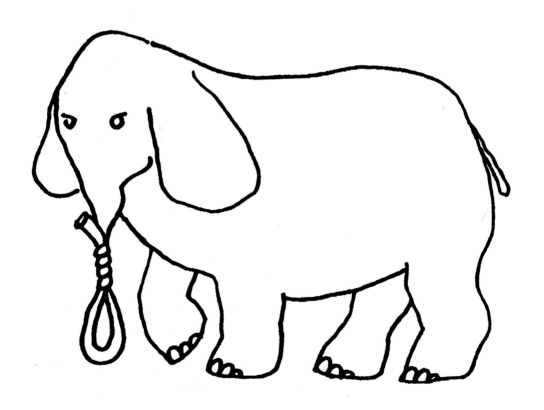

IMPEACHMENT

IN CONGRESS.
The unanimous Declaration
JULY 4. 1776.
States of America.

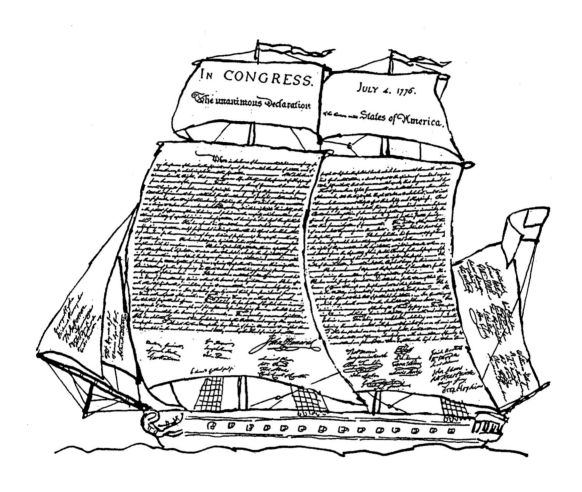

SHIP OF STATE 1776

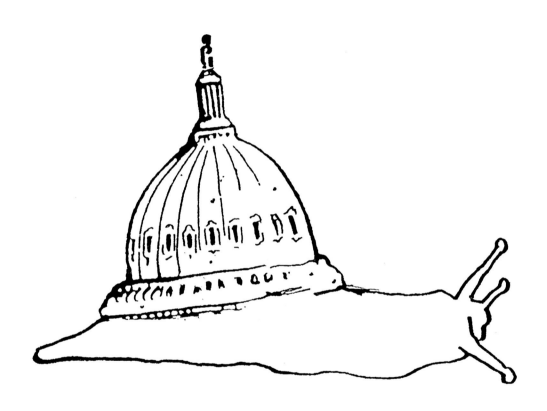

CONGRESS

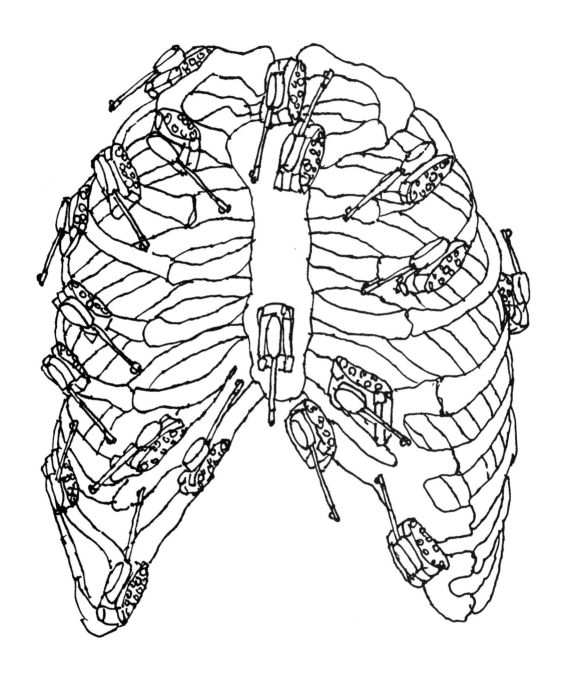

BAGHDAD ROADMAP

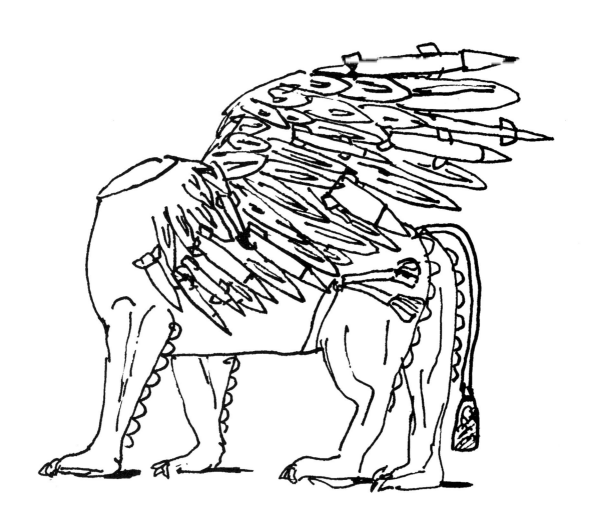

ON THE DEATH OF ZARQAWI

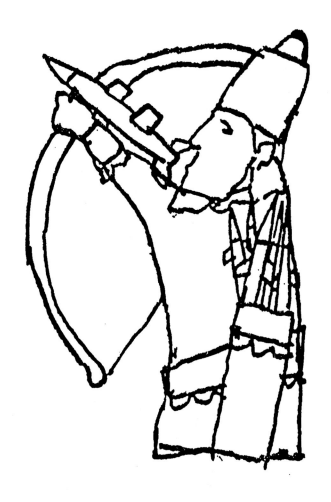

INSURGENCY

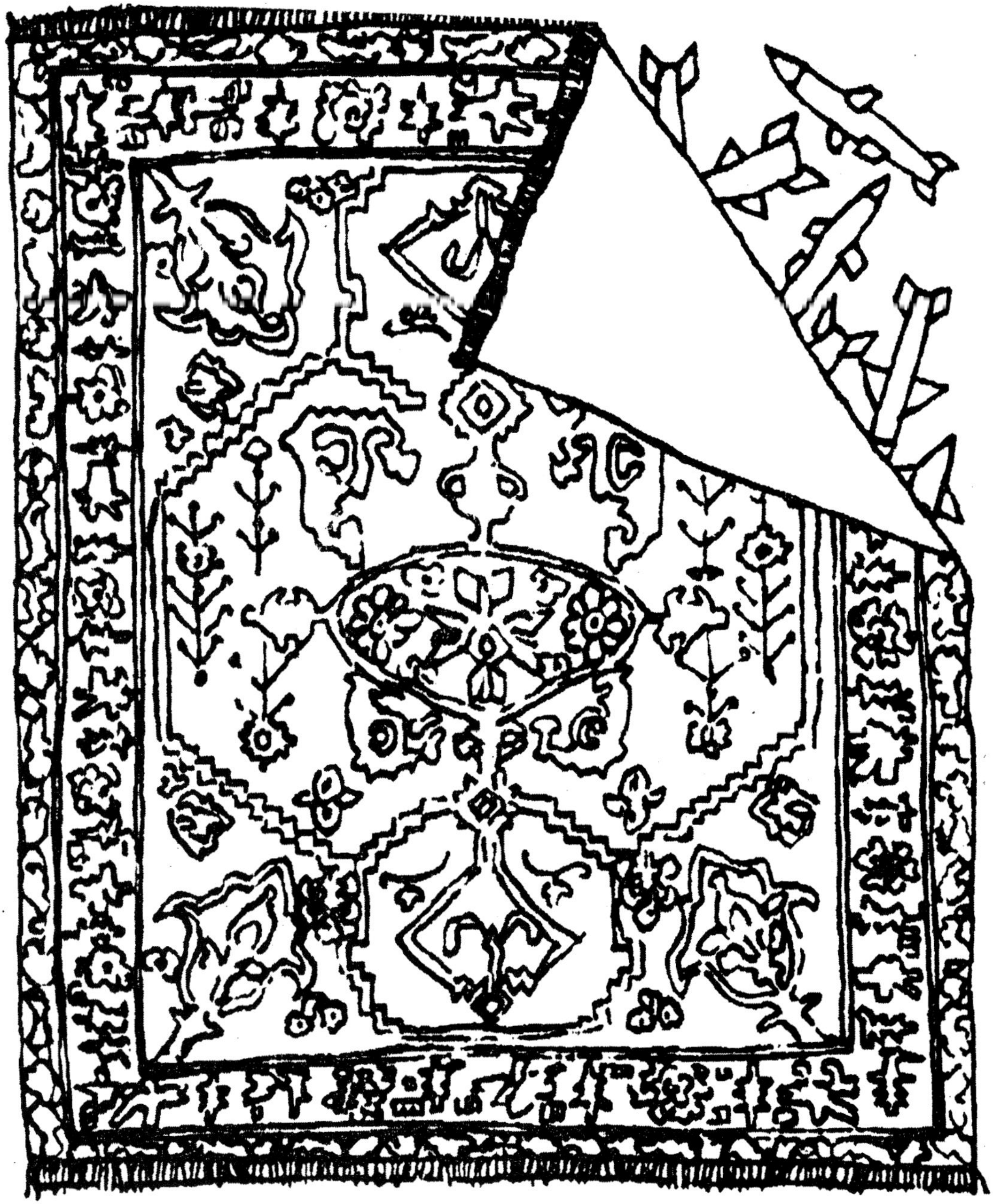

Iran

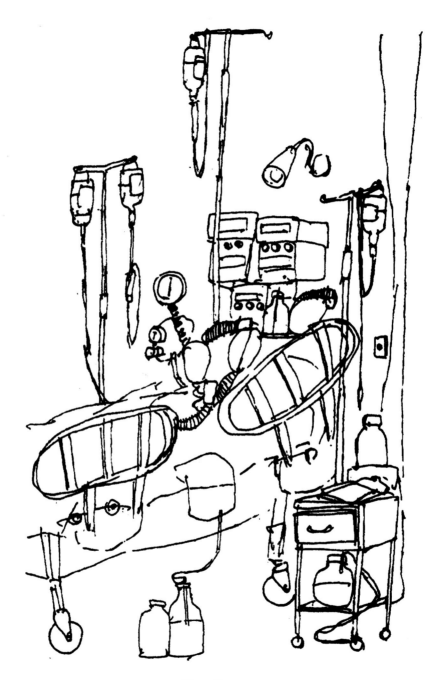

THE END

ACKNOWLEDGMENTS

It was my friend and colleague Dr. A. Bernard Ackerman who initially conceived the idea of publishing a collection of my drawings on medical subjects. Erika Goldman and Dr. Jerome Lowenstein of Bellevue Literary Press have been enthusiastic about this book from the moment the concept was presented to them. I am honored to have an introduction written by my classmate and friend Dr. Walter Reich. My son Michael's thoughtful suggestions were of immense value. Distinguished designers, among them Louise Fili and Bernard Schleifer, only make my art look better. Many of the drawings, which first appeared in *The New York Times,* were commissioned by art directors Jerelle Kraus and Steve Heller. Robert and Cheryl Fishko have elegantly exhibited my works at their prestigious Forum Gallery.

While a third year student at New York University School of Medicine, Dean Martin Begun gave me my first one-person exhibition, which was held in Alumni Hall. At the time, Dr. Adrian Zorgniotti introduced me to David Levine, described by Jules Feiffer as "the best social political literary caricaturist of this century." After looking at my drawings, David inscribed one of his books for me with the words: "Me, I'm a tennis player; You, you're no doctor. Draw!"

For the forty years since then, I have.